Eighteen Spa Smoothies and Juices

To Look and Feel Your Best

By Natasha Ross

Another amazing Healthy Smoothie and juice recipe book, from life coach and spa owner Natasha Ross. Natasha has been helping her clients to lose weight for many years. Now you can look and feel your best with some of the same organic smoothie and juice recipes that she has created for her clients, an amazing yet simple recipe book, with all natural ingredients to help you stay healthy all day. You can enjoy these smoothies anytime of the day. Drink to your health!!!

Copyright © 2020 Natasha Ross. All rights reserved.
Published by Natasha Ross.
ISBN 978-1-71699-032-8

Table of Contents

Before we get started

You will need:

- Measuring spoons
- A Knife or vegetable peeler
- A Chopping board
- A Colander
- Alkaline Water
- Juicer
- Blender or Nutribullet

A few tips:

Pre wash all fruits and vegetables before you begin, be sure to use organic if you can.

Chop ingredients into chunks. Use the blender at a low speed so your blender's heat will not destroy the healthy benefits in the fruits and vegetables. Try your best to get pure liquids for your smoothies, keep it organic.

Eighteen Spa Smoothies and Juices

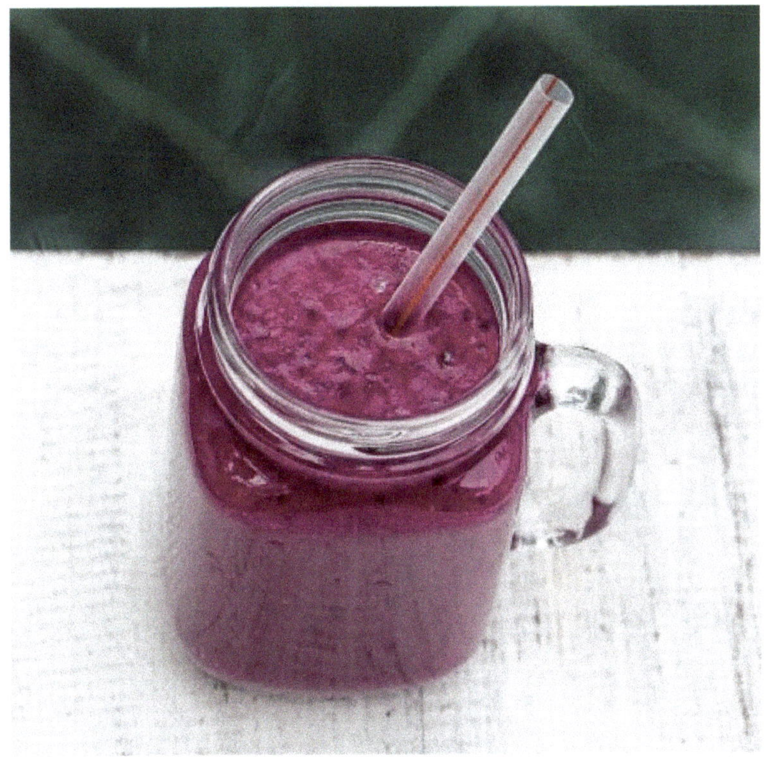

By

Natasha Ross

Blueberry Banana Strawberry Smoothie

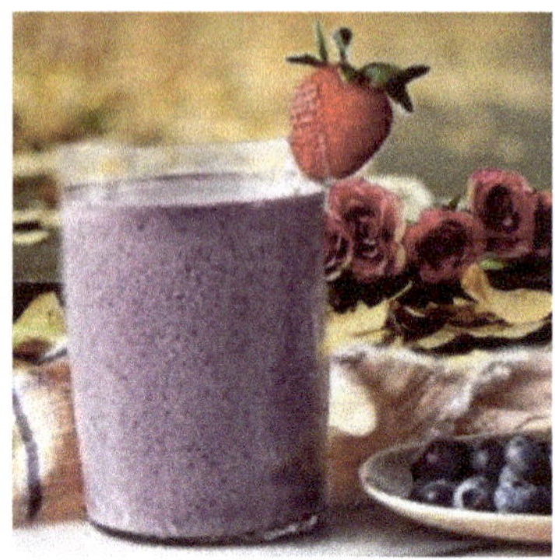

Ingredients:
- Feel free to use fresh or frozen fruits in your smoothies.
- I only add ice cubes if I am not using frozen fruits
- 1/2 cup of blueberries
- 1 cup of strawberries
- 2 bananas
- 1 ½ cup hemp or coconut milk (alkaline water optional)
- 2 tablespoons of sea moss (optional)
- 1 tbsp of agave (optional)
- 1 cup ice cubes (optional)
- Pinch of cinnamon

Be sure to wash your blueberries and strawberries before using.

Directions:
- In your blender or smoothie maker
- Add the hemp milk,
- Strawberries, blueberries, banana's
- Sea moss
- Cinnamon
- Agave
- Ice cubes

Blend on high until you get the smooth consistency you desire
Pour into beautiful glasses and enjoy. If you are allergic to any of these ingredients please substitute it for something else.

Great Juice For The Entire Family

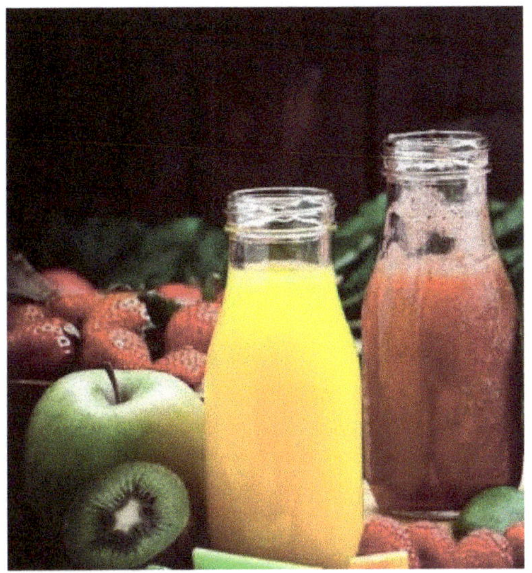

Ingredients:
- 2 Cups of Coconut Water or Alkaline Water
- 2 Carrots
- 2 Celery Stalks
- 1 Beet
- 2 Green Apples
- ½ Lemon squeezed
- 3 Inch of Ginger Peeled
- 3 Inches Turmeric Peeled

Directions

Please wash all of your Vegetables before use, and use organic if you can.

Chop into desired pieces and put into your juicer or blender, blend to your desired smoothness Pour into a beautiful glass and enjoy.

It is healthy and refreshing.

Spinach-Kale Berry Smoothie

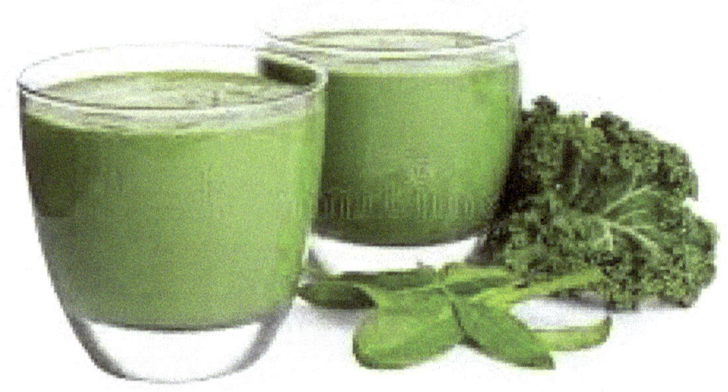

Ingredients:
- 1 cup spinach
- 1 cup kale
- 1 handful blackberries
- 1/2 cup raspberries
- 2 cups coconut water, or alkaline water
- 1 cup Kiwi
- 2-3 tablespoon sea moss
- 1 cups of ice cubes

Directions

In your Smoothie Maker/blender add Spinach and Kale with coconut water blend for 10 seconds on high Then add kiwi, blackberries, raspberries sea moss and ice cubes Blend until smooth.

Pour and serve. When I am making this smoothie drink with my family and friends I don't add maple syrup to my own but my friends do put maple syrup in their smoothies and that's okay, some people like sweets and some don't.

Pineapple Berry Ginger Coconut Smoothie

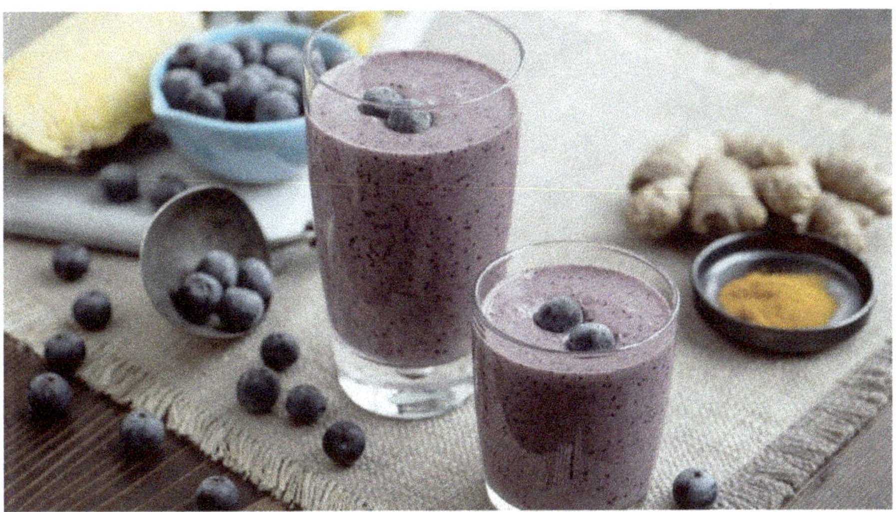

Ingredients:

- 1 ½ cup of coconut milk or flax milk
- 1 cup of organic strawberries
- 1 cup of organic raspberries
- 1 cup of golden berries (optional)
- 1 cup of chopped pineapples
- 1 inch of fresh ginger (optional)
- 1 tbsp of chia seeds
- 1 tbsp flax seeds
- 1 cup of ice cubes
- 2 tbsp of organic maple syrup (optional)
- 1/4 tablespoon of organic vanilla extract (optional)

If you are not using frozen fruits, add 1-2 cups of Ice cubes made with Alkaline or filtered water.

Directions:

In a blender or smoothie maker add the coconut milk
Next add the remaining ingredients, blend to a smooth consistency.
Serve in desired glasses and garnish with a few slices of strawberries or pineapples.

Cool Purple Punch

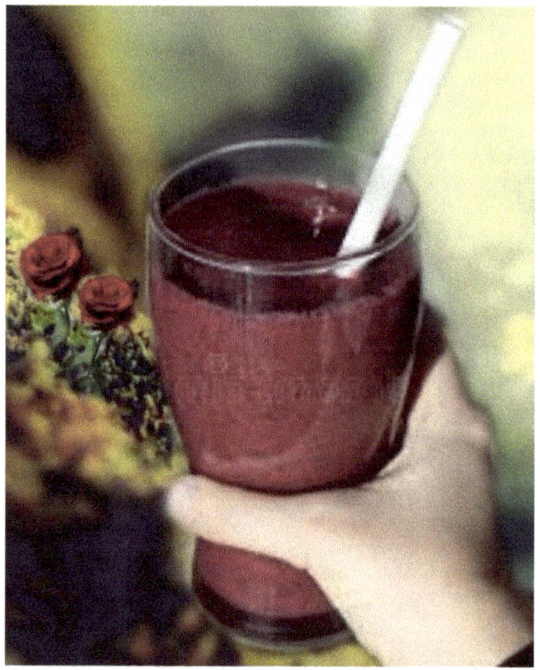

Ingredients:
- 1 Cup of Organic blueberries
- 1 Beetroot peeled and chopped
- 2 cups of coconut water or alkaline water
- 8 ounce of organic raspberry lemonade (optional)
- 2 purple carrots
- 3 Figs
- 1 Tablespoons of Flax seeds
- 1 Tablespoons of Chia seeds (optional)
- 4 tbsp of sea moss

Directions

Combine Coconut water and all other ingredients in your blender until well blended, strain with a juice mesh strainer and pour into desired glass and enjoy and drink to your health.

Blueberry Banana Spinach Sea moss Smoothie

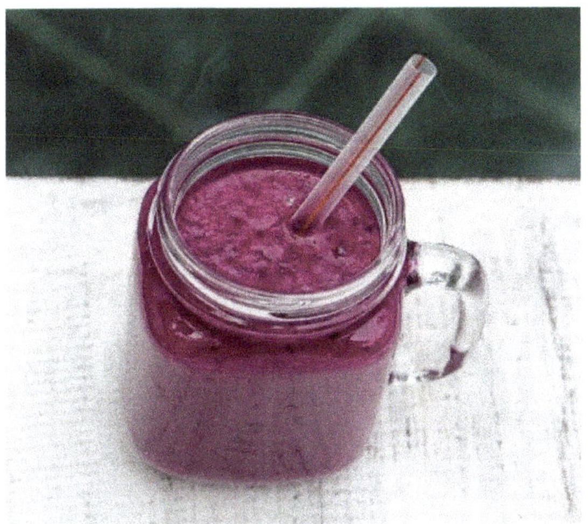

Ingredients:
- 2 ½ Cups of coconut water
- 2 Handfuls of Organic Spinach
- 1 Cup of plain or organic yogurt
- 1 Cup of Organic Blueberries
- ½ Cup blackberries
- 1 Organic Banana
- 1.5 Cup of chopped Pineapples
- 3 to 4 Mint Leaves

Directions

Pour the coconut water into smoothie maker then add the spinach blend and then add the yogurt and all other fruits and mix to a very smooth consistency

Pour and enjoy.

When I make this smoothie I treat myself as if I am at a five star restaurant or a spa, by pouring it into a beautiful glass garnish with extra mint leaves and a straw.

Banana Strawberry Almond Smoothie

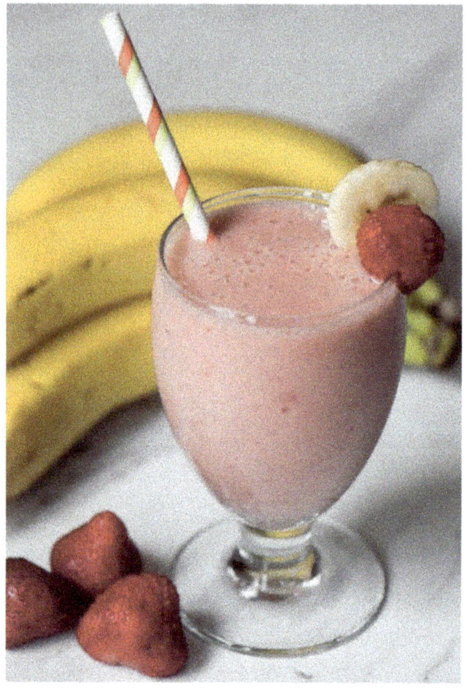

Ingredients

- 4 tablespoons of almond butter
- 2 organic Bananas
- 6 organic Strawberries
- 1 ½ cups almond milk
- 2 tablespoon of sea moss
- 1 cups Ice Cubes (optional)
- Sweeten to taste with maple syrup if desired
- Organic vanilla Extract (optional)

Directions

Place all of your ingredients into a blender and Blend into a smooth creamy mixture. Pure and enjoy.

Pistachio Pumpkin Banana Smoothie

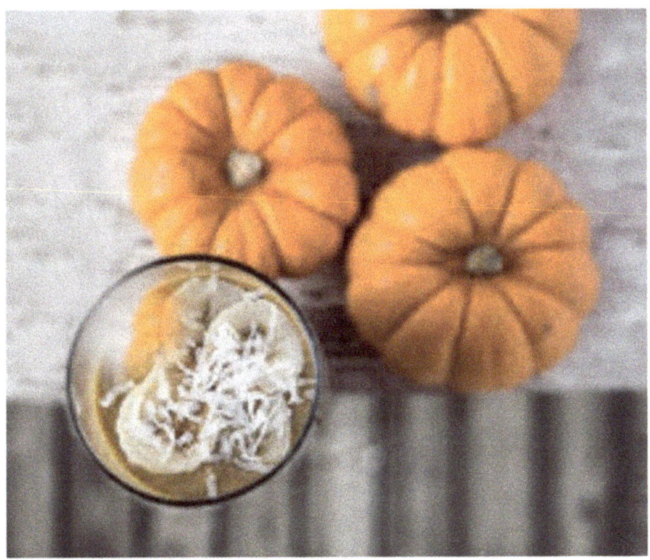

Ingredients

- 1 cup of hemp milk
- 3-4 tablespoons of hemp yogurt
- 1 tablespoon of sea moss
- 1-2 tablespoon of maple syrup (optional)
- 1 banana
- 1/4 cup pistachios
- 1/4 teaspoon cinnamon
- 1/2 cup ice cubes (optional)
- 1 cup of pumpkin cubed or puree
- 1 tbsp sea moss (Optional)

Directions:

Add all the ingredients in a blender

Pulse until well blended.

Pour and serve enjoy with a sprinkle of Cinnamon and a straw (optional)

Strawberry flaxseed Banana smoothie

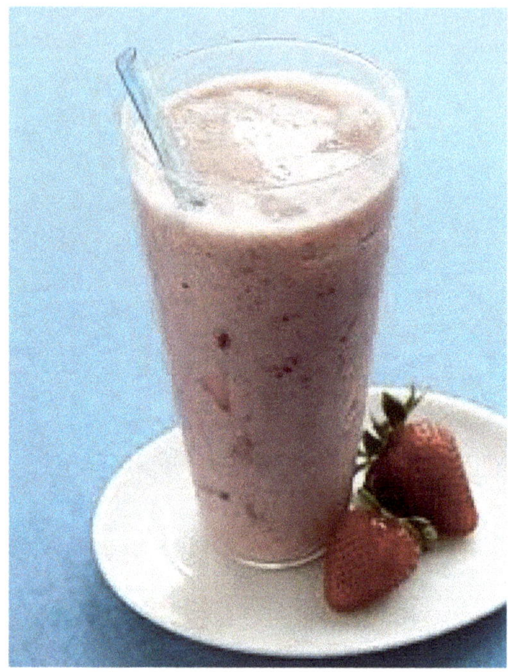

Ingredients:
- 1 ½ Cup of Almond or coconut milk
- 2 Cups of plain yogurt
- 2 Cups of Organic strawberries
- 3 Organic bananas
- 4 tbsp of Organic honey
- 1 tbsp of flax seeds
- 1 tbsp of hemp seeds
- 1 tbps sea moss
- 1 Cup of Ice cubes (Optional)

Directions

Pour milk into blender and add all of the other ingredients and blend well.

Serve and enjoy cold

Moringa Apple Kiwi Smoothie

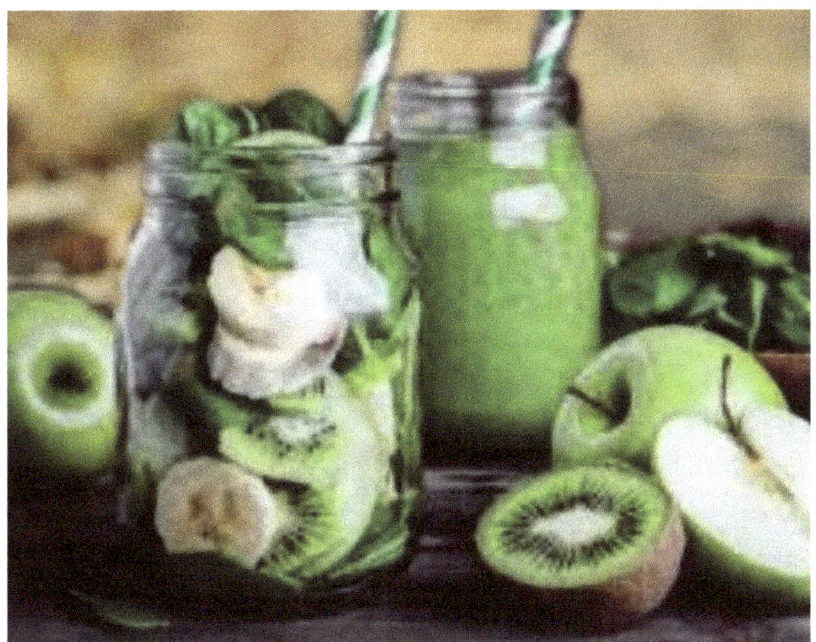

Ingredients:
- 2 Cups of Coconut Water
- 3 Organic Celery Stalks
- 2 Organic Apples
- 1 Organic Kiwi
- 1 Handful Of Organic Green Grapes
- 4 Mint Leaves
- 1 tsp of Moringa Powder
- 1 Cups Of Ice Cubes. (optional)
- 1 tbps sea moss

Directions

Put coconut water in the blender add celery and blend then add the other ingredients and blend until smooth

This is a very good pick me upper in the morning

Coconut Yogurt Cantaloupe Smoothie

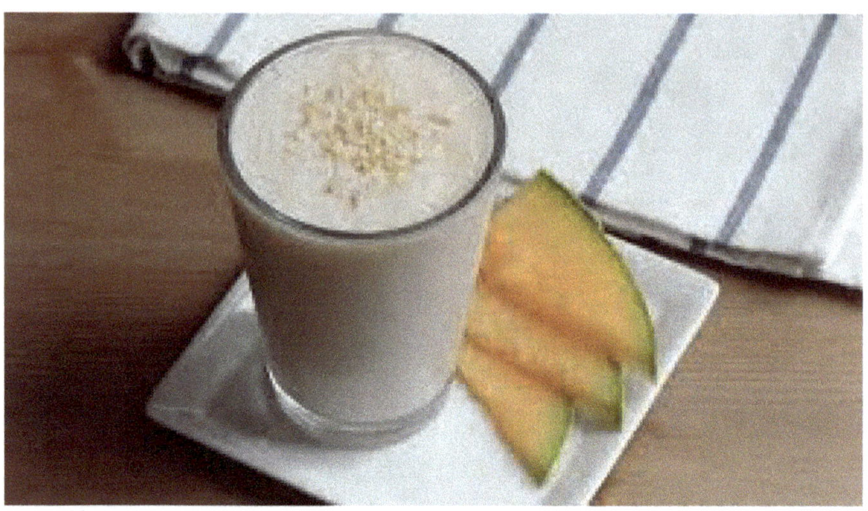

Ingredients:

- 2 Cups coconut milk (or milk of your choice)
- 1 ½ Cup Organic Coconut Yogurt
- 2 ½ Cups of Cantaloupe (cut into chunks)
- 1 Organic Avocado
- 6 Mint Leaves
- I Tablespoon hemp seeds
- 2 Cups Crushed Ice
- Add some agave to sweeten (optional)

Directions

In a blender combine all ingredients until well blended and serve.

Mango Kale Swiss Chard Smoothie

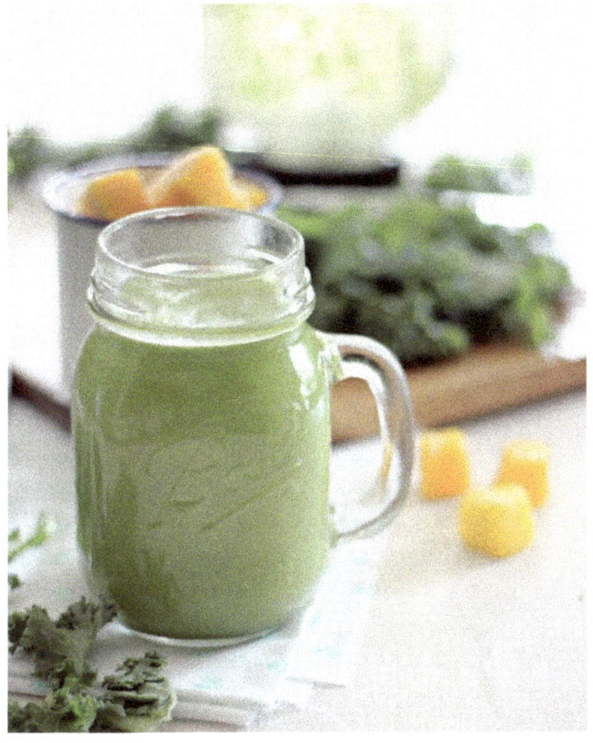

Ingredients:
- 2 Cups of coconut milk
- 1 Handful of Kale
- 1 Mango peeled and diced
- I Banana
- 1 Handful of Swiss chard
- 1 tbsp of maca powder
- Agave to sweeten to desired sweetness (optional)
- 1 tbsp flax seed (optional)
- 2 Cups crushed ice

Directions

Combine coconut milk and kale and swiss chard in the blender
then stop the blender and add the other ingredients blend well, enjoy.

Spinach Avocado Maca Root Smoothie

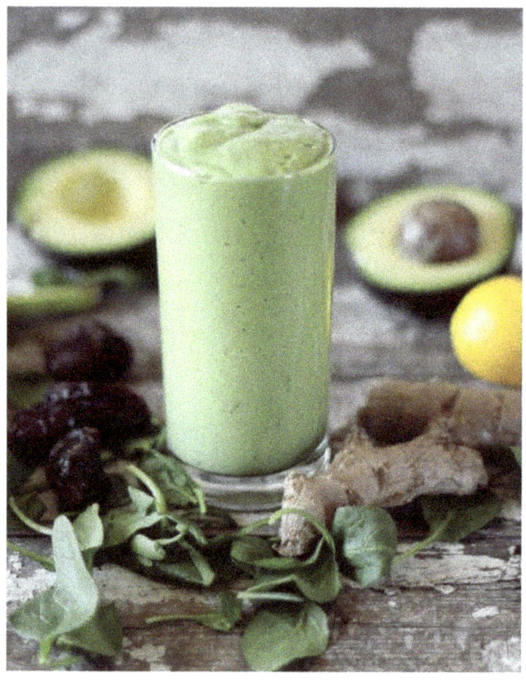

Ingredients

- 2 Cups of almond milk
- 2 Handful of fresh organic spinach
- 2 Cups of crushed ice avocado
- 1 Banana
- 1 Mango
- 2 tbsp of maca root powder
- 4-6 tbsp of maple syrup
- 1-2 Cups or Ice

Directions

Add almond milk and spinach in the blender blend then add your other ingredients and blend well

Pour into desired glasses and garnish with a sprinkle of cinnamon and a couple of cinnamon sticks.

Strawberry Pineapple Chia Smoothie

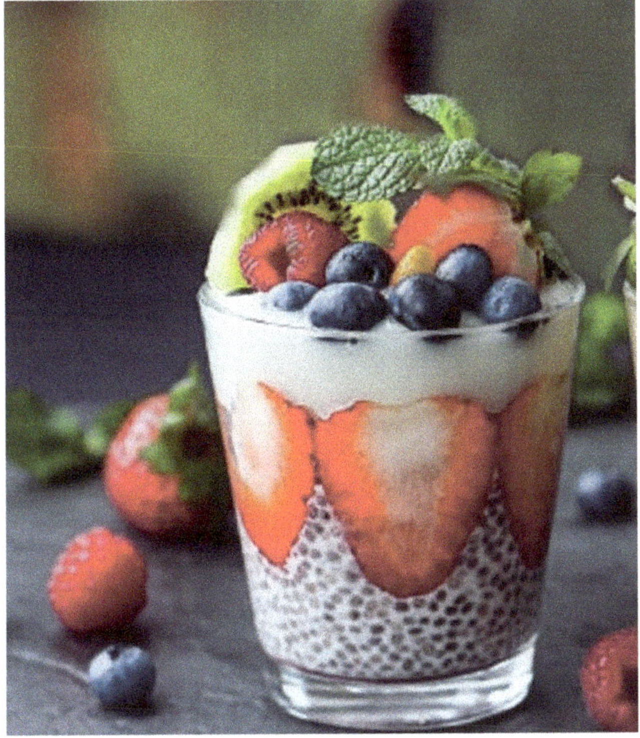

Ingredients:
- 1 Cup of Alkaline water
- 2 Cups of Organic Strawberries (fresh or frozen)
- 1/2 Cup of diced Pineapples
- 1 Cup of carrot Juice
- 1 tbsp Chia seed (optional)
- Maple syrup (optional)
- 1 tbsp sea moss (optional)

Directions

Pour the milk into your blender and then add all other ingredients and blend

Serve and enjoy!

Your All Veggie Smoothie

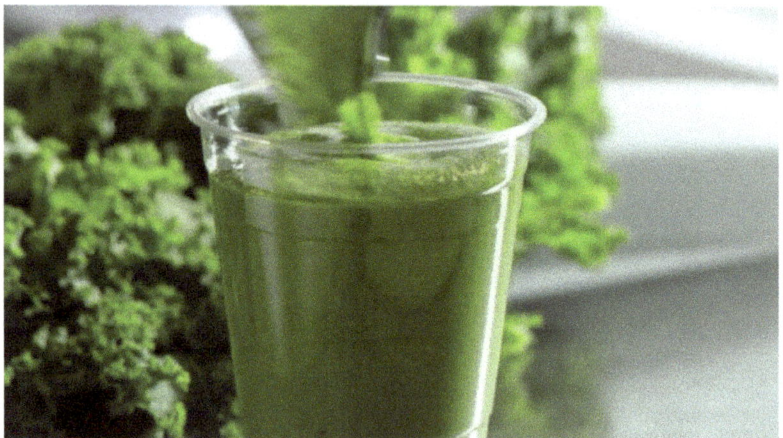

My Favorite all time veggie smoothie, I have this twice a week after my workouts or I take it along with me on my walks. You can have this drink at any time. Try organic vegetables if you can.

Ingredients:
- 3-4 Cups of coconut water, add more if needed (sometimes I just use alkaline water)
- 2 Cups of greens (I just use whatever I have at that time)
- 1/4 Cup parsley
- 2 Celery stalks organic
- 1/2 of a small onion
- 1/2 Red bell pepper
- 1/2 Green bell pepper
- 1/2 Zucchini
- 1/2 Cucumber
- 1/2 tbsp kelp powder (optional)

Directions

In the nutribullet or blender combine the water, the greens and the parsley blend and follow with all of the ingredients and blend well.

Carrot goodness

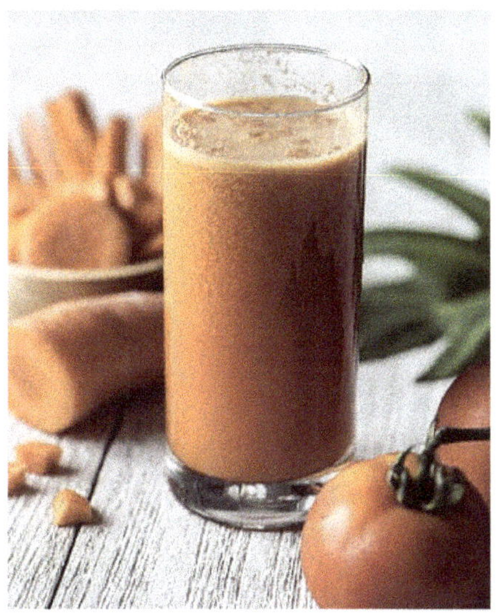

Ingredients:

- 1 cup of coconut water
- 4 Large Organic carrots
- 1 Cup chopped peaches
- 2 Organic granny smith apples
- 3 Inch piece of ginger root
- 2 inch piece of turmeric
- ½ fresh lemon juice
- 1 tbsp sea moss (optional)

Directions:

- Wash your fruits and spice roots
- Chop into chunks and feed through your juicer
- You can also add 2 cups of alkaline water to your smoothie maker or blender
- Add the carrots, then your ginger and turmeric roots, followed by your granny smith apples, blend well.
- Pour into a glass and enjoy with or without Ice.
- Turmeric has great potent anti - inflammatory benefits

My Womb Smoothie

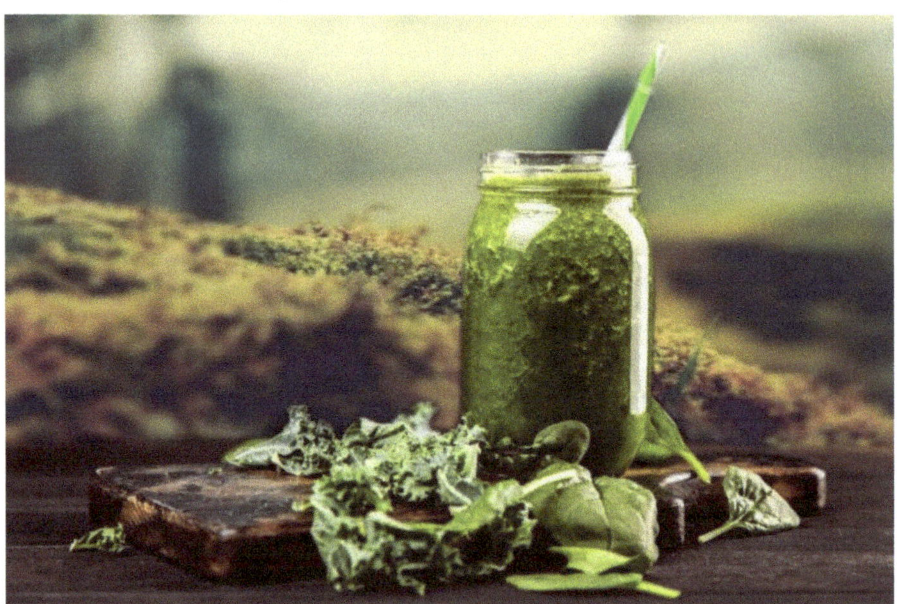

Ingredients

- 2 cups coconut water or alkaline water
- 1 cup spinach,
- 1 cup lettuce
- 1 cup kale
- 1 cup Broccoli
- ½ Avocado
- 1 pear
- ½ fresh lime juice (optional)
- 1 cup ice

Directions:

Put all of your ingredients into your blender or nutribullet or blender and until smooth and serve chilled

Papaya Skin Glow

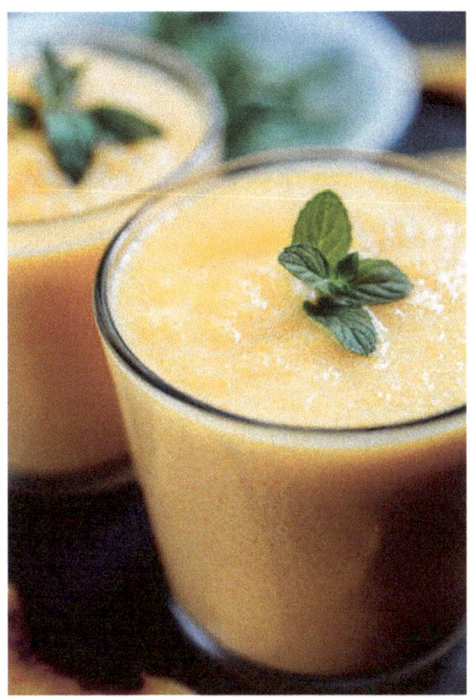

Ingredient

- 1 ¼ cups fresh or frozen ripe papaya
- 1 small ripe banana (previously peeled, sliced and frozen)
- 1 tsp turmeric
- 1 tbsp lime juice
- 1/2 cup carrot juice
- 1 cup ice (optional)
- 1 cup coconut water or milk of you choice depending on your health need

Directions:

Place all ingredients into a blender and blend until smooth

Pour into a cup and serve

Strawberry's Benefits

- Boosts the immune system
- Maintain normal blood pressure
- Minimizes risk of Cancer and arthritis
- Help by reducing eye related ailments
- It also has the potential to regulate our nervous system
- Strawberries can prevent heart diseases while reducing cholesterol.

Blueberries Benefits

- Helps with Alzheimer's disease
- Prevents signs of aging.
- Reduces the risk of macular degeneration, cataracts and myopia
- Aids in the prevention of dementia
- Boosts immune system function
- Helps by preventing Hair loss and Osteoporosis
- Help prevent urinary tract infection
- Improves digestion while providing relief from constipation

Apple Benefits

- Weight loss
- Digestion
- Controls blood sugar levels
- Lowers cholesterol levels
- Improves eyesight

- Prevents cancer
- Treats anemia

Cucumber Benefits

- Weight loss
- Manages diabetes
- Help with constipation
- Brightening of the skin
- Lowers blood pressure
- Reduces risk of kidney stones

Watermelon Benefits

- Lowers blood pressure
- Lowers blood sugar elves in diabetics
- Effective in helping with erectile dysfunction
- Prevents heat strokes
- Reduces the risk of kidney disorder
- Eye health
- Repairs tissue in the body

Pineapple Benefits

- Improves eye and oral health
- Helps with arthritis, cancer, heart disease
- Boots immunity, improves blood circulation
- Irritable bowel syndrome and constipation
- Reduces inflammation in the joints

- Helps by reducing risk of dementia
- Alzheimer's disease

Avocado Benefits

- Maintains healthy Skin
- Assist with weight digestion and weight management
- Reduces risk of cardiovascular disease
- Keep eyes healthy
- Helps with vitamin K deficiency
- Protects the liver
- Prevents bad breath

Figs Benefits

- Vision health
- Respiratory health
- Digestion
- Weight management
- Sexual health
- Strengthens bones
- Lowers cholesterol
- Increases fertility
- Protects the heart
- Regulates kidney and liver function
- Lower blood pressure
- Lower incidences of macular degeneration, and inhibits some cancers

Kiwi Benefits

- Reduces risk of eye related ailments
- Rich in antioxidants
- Boosts immune system
- Lowers risk of diabetes and cancer
- Beneficial for fetal development
- Maintain healthy cardiovascular system

Mango Benefits

- Can prevent Cancers
- Boosts the immune system
- Improves digestion
- Helps to fight heat strokes
- Improves yes health
- Lowers cholesterol
- Alkalizes the whole body
- It's also a great sauce of vitamin C
- May help with diabetes

Raspberries Benefits

- Helps with weight loss
- Regulates menstrual cycle in women
- Reduces wrinkles and age spots
- Reduces risk of macular degeneration
- Boosts immunity and protects against cancer
- Relieves nausea in pregnant women
- Helps in boosting milk in lactating mothers

Banana Benefits

- Protects against ulcers
- Kidney disorders
- Reduces menstrual problems
- Provides relief from constipation
- Can also help with hemorrhoids and anemia
- It may give some relief from arthritis and gout

Cantaloupe Benefits

- Improves insulin metabolism
- Prevents kidney related diseases
- Protects the against toxins and premature aging
- Maintains healthy eyes
- Boosts immunity and prevents cancer
- Reduces inflammation and prevents arthritis

Golden Berries Benefits

- Help to maintain optimal liver, kidney and heart health
- Protects against chronic diseases and cancer
- Boots immune system and coronary heart diseases
- Aids in weight loss and managing diabetes
- Reduces risk of atherosclerosis and coronary heart diseases
- Also beneficial in maintaining lower levels of bad cholesterol

Grapes Benefits

- Help cure asthma and migraine
- Effective remedy against breast cancer
- Prevent heart attacks and lowers cholesterol
- Strengthens bones and prevent onset of osteoporosis
- Relief from constipation and indigestion
- Boosts immune system and prevents fatigue
- Vision and brain function

Blackberries Benefits

- It is said that it improves and maintain brain function
- Reduce inflammation, fights infection and boosts immunity
- Regulates menstrual health
- Great for the cardiovascular system
- Promotes skin health
- May also prevent cancer growth

Celery Benefits

- Helps to relief asthma and bronchitis symptoms
- Cleanses the kidney
- Relieves arthritis
- Lowers high blood pressure

Kale Benefits

- Cancer prevention
- Antioxidant
- Detoxification
- Vision health
- Brain development in infants
- Supports the Heart
- Anti - Inflammatory

Swiss Chard Benefits

- Very high in antioxidants
- Help in protecting eye health
- Bone health
- Protects heart health
- Helps prevent diabetes
- Helps with maintaining brain function
- Slows the aging process
- Digestion improves
- Fights cancer

Spinach Benefits

- Protects against cancer
- Boosts immunity
- Defends against heart disease
- Eye health
- Helps maintain bone health
- Skin health

- Brain health

Onion Benefits

- Improves immunity
- Regulates blood sugar
- Reduces inflammation
- May Prevent cancer
- Reduces risk of gastric ulcers
- Lowers bad cholesterol

Kelp Benefits

- Great source of iodine
- Helps with detoxification
- Improves digestive health
- Help to control blood sugar
- It has anti - Inflammatory properties
- Thyroid health
- Lowers cholesterol

Carrots Benefits

- Improves eyesight
- Prevents heart diseases
- Reduces high blood pressure
- Maintains good digestive health
- Boots immune system
- Regulates blood sugar levels
- Prevents macular degeneration

- Reduces risk of cancer and strokes

Ginger Benefits

- Reduces risk of cancer
- Help cure nausea
- Provides menstrual cramp relief
- Boosts bone health and relieves joint pain
- Builds appetite and facilitates digestion
- Regulates high sugar levels

Parsley Benefits

- Prevents cancer
- Manages diabetes
- Boosts immune system
- Relief from rheumatoid arthritis
- Helps to control urinary tract infection and gallstone
- Protects against osteoporosis and improves bone health
- Reduces internal inflammation and helps to cleanse liver

Beets Benefits

- Reduces birth defects
- Reduces macular degeneration
- Prevents respiratory ailments
- Boosts immune system and heart health
- Prevents skin, lung and colon cancer
- Stimulates liver function

Pumpkin Benefits

- Promotes fertility and immune function
- Promotes eye health
- Promotes against asthma and heart disease
- Delays aging
- May lower blood pressure
- May reduce the risk of developing certain types of cancer
- Regulates high sugar levels

Bell Pepper Benefits

- Promotes healthy pregnancy
- Weight loss
- Supports eye health
- Reduces risk of cancer and heart disease
- Improves immunity
- Helps you to maintain good mental health
- Promotes healthy glowing skin

Zucchini Benefits

- Help in treating benign prostatic hypertrophy in men
- Gives relief from aching symptoms of rheumatoid arthritis
- Beneficial to weight loss
- Helps maintain optimal health
- Protects against infections and diseases
- Prevents cancer and cardiovascular diseases

Lemon Benefits

- Cures digestion
- May prevent cancer
- Treats rheumatism and arthritis
- Controls high blood pressure
- Offers relief from fever and cold
- Reduce weight
- Boosts immune system

Turmeric Benefits

- Boost cognitive abilities helps by reducing stress and depression
- Detoxifies the body, useful for treating gastrointestinal disorders
- Beneficial in maintaining healthy heart
- Rich in anti-inflammatory properties
- Relieve menstrual pain and gives relief from fatigue nausea, pelvic pain and cramps,
- Cancer treatment and prevention

Maca Benefits

- Boost immune system, rich in antidepressant properties
- Improve sexual stamina and drive
- Helps to increase bone density and strength
- Promotes homeostasis or balance within the body
- Increase sperm count and motility of men

- Reduces anxiety and mood swings in postmenopausal women

Flax Seed Benefits

- Flax seed helps the digestive system
- Fights breast, prostate, ovarian and colon cancer
- High in omega-3 fatty acids
- Have shown to have benefits for menopausal women
- High in antioxidants, flax seeds are gluten-free
- Lowers cholesterol, supports weight loss
- Promotes healthy skin and hair
- High in fiber

Hemp Seeds Benefits

- Hemp seeds aids in digestion,
- Boost immune system,
- Provides relief from insomnia and strengthens bones
- Beneficial in weight management
- Helps to prevent anemia and headaches
- Helps to cure diarrhea and constipation

Chia seeds Benefits

- Controls hypertension, lowers cholesterol levels, prevent heart diseases
- Help with weight management
- Boost gastrointestinal health, prevents calcium deficiency

- Prevents fatigue, helps to control diabetes
- Prevents arthritis

Mint leaves Benefits

- Promotes digestion health
- Improves oral health
- Helps to prevent cancer
- Quick and effective remedy for nausea
- Clears up congestion of nose, throat and lungs
- Natural stimulant, relieves from fatigue and depression

Moringa Benefits

- Moringa treats edema, protects liver
- Treat stomach disorders, great for skin and hair care
- Acts as antibacterial agents
- Cures cancer, treats Nero degenerative diseases, improve bone health
- Boost immunity, protects cardiovascular system, treats diabetes, treats asthma Protects against Stone formation,
- Protects against kidney problems
- Has antifertility effects
- Heals wound
- Reduces hypertension
- Improve eye health
- Treats anemia and sickle cell disease

Pistachios Benefits

- Pistachios boost immune system
- Gives relief from constipation
- Improves metabolism
- Reduces risk of heart attack and strokes
- Provides wound healing and cellular growth
- Beneficial for digestion and intestinal health
- Defense against diabetes

Facts:

- Sea Moss has 92 of the 102 minerals that our bodies need.

- It promotes a healthy thyroid.

- It also works as a booster on the immune system.

- It provides better circulation.

- It's rich in vitamins and minerals, to name a few:

- vitamin-C and B, magnesium, manganese, sulfur, potassium, calcium, selenium, iodine, protein, phosphorus, bromine, zinc, beta-carotene, pectin.

- Sea Moss is great for adults and children. I grew up on sea moss, everyday my mom prepared it for us when we got home from a long day at school.

Eighteen Spa Smoothies and Juices

To Look and Feel Your Best

By Natasha Ross

www.ingramcontent.com/pod-product-compliance
Lightning Source LLC
Chambersburg PA
CBHW040806260726

48664CB00029B/1658